Preface

Current Asthma treatment consist mainly of inhaled Asthma medications available in several inhaler types, including pressurized Metered Dose Inhalers (pMDIs) and Dry Powder Inhalers (DPIs). The inhalation route delivers the drug directly to the airways; the dose required is smaller than when given by mouth and side effects are reduced.

Many Asthma patients derive incomplete benefits from their inhaled medication because they do not use their inhaler devices correctly, or they fail to maintain the correct inhaler technique. The Global initiative for Asthma (GINA) suggests that, the correct use of inhalers is an important feature in preventing exacerbations of Asthma.

Informing patients about their Asthma could help in achieving better control over their Asthma symptoms in addition; Asthma patients need to be trained, on the correct use of their prescribed inhaler devices.

The text begins with an introduction to Asthma and a description of the major pharmacological groups of medicines normally used in Asthma inhalers. The various types of inhalers are described. The text concludes with patient education and inhaler training section in addition to self- assessment section.

This text may be of interest to Asthma nurse, pharmacy technician, pharmacist, or a doctor.
M.A.Qarawi
BSc, Mphil, PhD, GPhC

Contents

1-Introduction to Asthma

Asthma is a chronic inflammatory disorder of the airways. The word Asthma originates from an ancient Greek word meaning panting hyperactive response (also called hyper responsiveness). The chronic inflammatory disorder in Asthma is associated with airway hyper-responsiveness (exaggerated response), to wide variety of allergic or non-allergic triggers, leading to airflow obstruction that is reversible.[2]

Asthma most commonly develops in early childhood, and more than three quarters of children who develop Asthma symptoms before the age of seven years, no longer have symptoms by the age of sixteen years.[2] However, Asthma can develop at any stage in life, including adulthood.

Admission to hospital during an Asthma attack may indicate the first episode in the disease, or failure of preventative care for established Asthma.

The respiratory tract

The respiratory tract or lungs comprise two conducting regions, upper and lower regions. The upper respiratory tract comprises the nose, throat, pharynx and larynx. The lower respiratory tract comprises the trachea, bronchi, bronchioles and the alveolar region (figure 1).

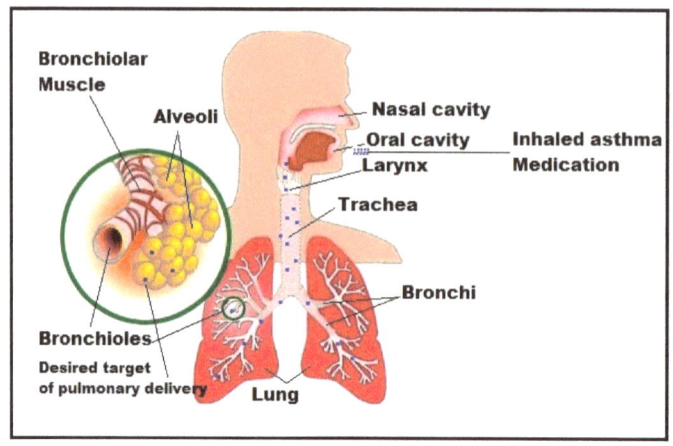

Fig 1. The respiratory tract

Oxygen and carbon dioxide are exchanged between blood and inhaled air in the alveolar region.

Asthma symptoms are believed to be due to tightening of muscles lining the bronchioles. The alveolar sacs are normally the target site for inhaled Asthma medications.

Asthma triggers

A trigger for Asthma in a patient is anything which starts Asthma symptoms or makes the Asthma symptoms worse in the patient, examples of Asthma triggers include physical exercise and outdoor air pollution, several examples of Asthma triggers are presented in table 1.

Dust mites	Dust mites are tiny bugs that are in almost every home. If you have Asthma, dust mites can trigger an Asthma attack.
Outdoor Air Pollution	Outdoor air pollution can trigger an Asthma attack. This pollution can come from factories, cars, and other sources.
Tobacco Smoke	Tobacco smoke is unhealthy for everyone, especially people with Asthma.
Cockroach Allergen	Cockroaches and their droppings can trigger an Asthma attack.
Other Triggers	Infections linked to influenza (flu), Colds, Allergy, Physical exercise and Some medicines such as Ibuprofen, propranolol can also trigger Asthma attack.

Table 1: Some common asthma triggers. [3]

The chronic inflammation in Asthma is associated with the airways exaggerated response to various allergic or non-allergic triggers, the airways exaggerated response can lead to recurrent episodes of wheezing, breathlessness, chest tightness, and coughing in affected individuals.

What triggers Asthma symptoms in one patient may be different to what triggers asthma in another patient. If patients understand which things trigger their asthma, they might be able to avoid them or seek medical help in order to get appropriate treatment in order to reduce the effects of Asthma triggers.

Asthma diagnosis

The diagnosis of Asthma should be made by a qualified clinician, diagnosing Asthma by a qualified clinician, normally involve taking a medical history of the patient, in addition to performing physical examination and lung function tests.

Objective assessments of lung function are considered necessary for the diagnosis of Asthma because medical history and physical examination are not considered reliable means of excluding other diagnoses or of characterizing the status of lung impairment.

Spirometry

Spirometry is the main lung function test, doctors or Asthma nurses generally use to diagnose Asthma in people 5 years or older.[3] A Spirometer is an apparatus for measuring the volume of air inspired and expired by the lungs.

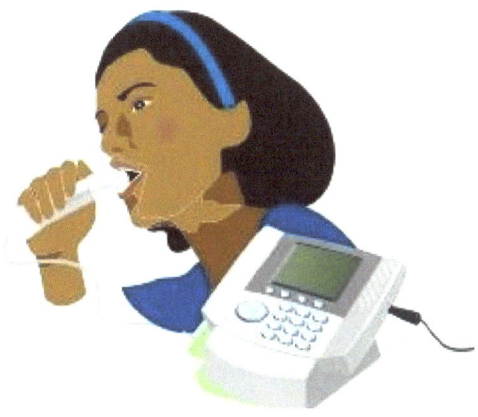

Fig 2. A Spirometer

The use of the spirometer involve taking a deep breath and forcibly breathing out (exhaling) into a tube connected to a spirometer. This records both the amount (volume) of air exhaled and how quickly it is exhaled. Spirometry typically measures the maximal volume of air forcibly exhaled from the point of maximal inhalation (FVC) and the volume of air exhaled during the first second and six seconds, FVC1 and FCV6 respectively, these tests are conducted before and after the patient inhales a short-acting bronchodilator. The test is normally undertaken for patients in whom the diagnosis of asthma is being considered, including children ≥5 years of age. These measurements help to determine whether there is airflow obstruction, its severity, and whether it is reversible over the short term.

Peak flow meters

A peak flow meter is a small hand-held device, used to measure how fast a patient can blow air out of their lungs in one breath, Peak Expiratory Flow (P.E.F). Peak flow meters are designed as monitoring, not as diagnostic, tools.

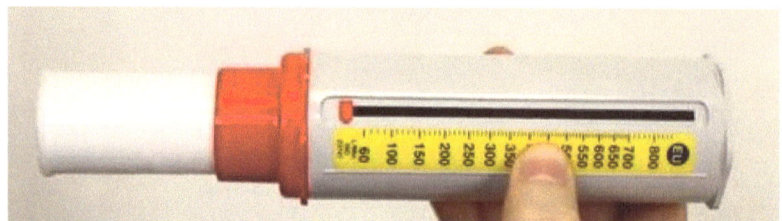

Fig 3. Peak flow meter, Mini-Wright brand, the mouthpiece is fitted on the device, and the marker is moved to zero prior to use by the patient.

Peak flow meters normally come in two ranges, a low-range peak flow meter is for small children and measures low peak expiratory flow rates, and a standard-range peak flow meter for older children, teenagers and adults. An adult has much larger airways than a child has and needs the larger range. There are several brands of peak flow meters. During the test the patient breathe in as deeply as they can and then blow into the peak flow meter as hard and fast as possible, P.E.F. is read from the device, normally several readings are taken at each occasion and the highest reading is recorded as one P.E.F. reading. If a person above five years of age is diagnosed with Asthma, they could be prescribed a peak flow meter to use at home. It can be used as a patient tool to assess the severity of Asthma, to check response to treatment or to monitor lung function when Asthma symptoms flare up in the patient, this help the clinician in recommending appropriate treatment.

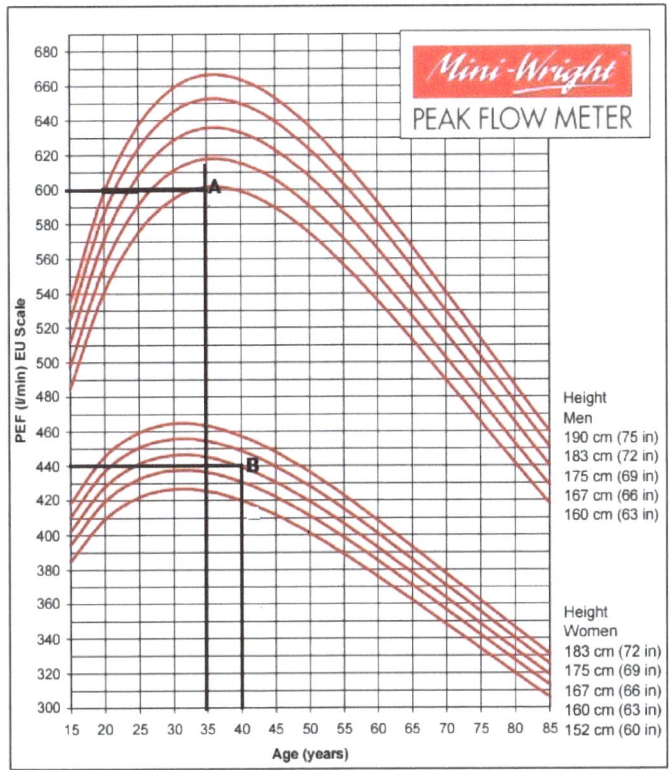

Adapted by Clement Clarke for use with EN13826 / EU scale peak flow meters
from Nunn AJ Gregg I, Br Med J 1989:298;1068-70

Fig 4. Peak flow charts show P.E.F for healthy people of different ages and physical characteristics, the charts are normally included with peak flow meters. For example: Point A on the chart represents the normal P.E.F (600 L/min) for a 35 year old male with a height of 160 cm, The normal P.E.F for a 40 year old female with a height of 167 cm is 440 L/min, as read from the peak flow chart point (B).

The P.E.F. charts of non-Asthmatics, with different ages, and physical characteristics, are useful for estimating the normal peak flow reading for Asthmatic patient.

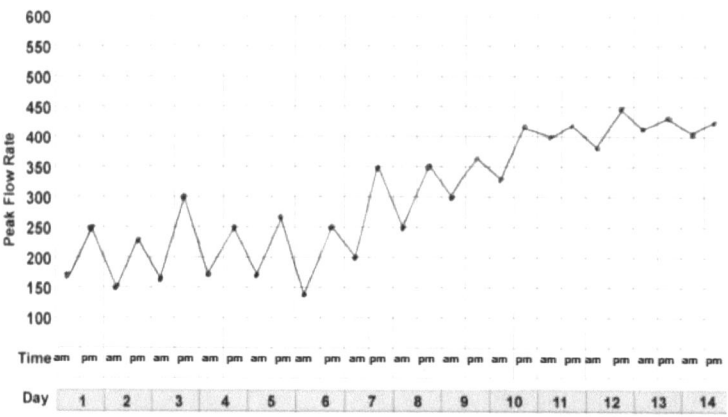

Fig 5. P.E.F readings for a patient, normally readings of a patient are taken twice daily and recorded on a blank chart, the blank chart is normally supplied with the peak flow meter.

For diagnostic purposes, spirometry is generally recommended over measurements by a peak flow meter because there is wide variability even in the published predicted peak expiratory flow (PEF) reference values. Reference values need to be specific to each brand of peak flow meter, and such normative brand-specific values currently are not available for most brands.[5]

2-Inhaled Asthma medications

Asthma normally requires ongoing management, as long as the Asthma condition exists. This includes using proper medication/s. Asthma medications can be given orally, parenterally or administration by inhalation (pulmonary drug delivery).

The use of inhaled medicines allows selective treatment of the lungs by achieving a high drug concentration in the airway while reducing systemic adverse effects. Aerosol drug delivery is painless and convenient. One of the most important disadvantages of aerosol therapy is that specific inhalation techniques are necessary for the proper use of each of the different available inhaler types. A less-than-optimal technique can result in decreased drug delivery and potentially reduced efficacy.

Inhaled Asthma medications are normally classified into the following groups according to their role in the management of asthma:

A- **Quick-relief medications (relievers)**

Quick-relief medications (relievers) are usually used to provide temporary relief of Asthma symptoms, reliever medications could also be used before exposure to a known asthma trigger such as exercise induced asthma attack. Relievers are normally bronchodilators, which help to open up the airways so that more air can flow through the lungs.

Two types of quick-relief medications are available;

I- Adrenoceptor agonists (sympathomimetics), Selective beta2 agonists produce bronchodilation. A short acting beta2 agonist is used for immediate relief of Asthma Symptoms, selective short acting $beta_2$ agonists include Salbutamol/albuterol and terbutaline. Short acting $beta_2$ agonists relax muscles around the bronchiole airways and provide prompt relief of asthma symptoms, normally they start to work within minutes and their therapeutic effect lasts for up to 4 hours. Everyone with a clinical diagnosis of Asthma should have a reliever medication.

A reliever inhaler is normally used when required, not on regular basis and may be used as preventer for exercise-induced asthma or before exposure to a known trigger/s. Reliever medications do not provide long-term Asthma control.

 The frequency of using a reliever medication is normally used by the prescriber, as one factor in assessing the need to review Asthma treatment, using standard protocols. Reference publications such as the most recent edition of the BNF or most recent guidelines of the American Thoracic Society; contain protocol for Asthma medication adjustments according to the severity of the Asthma condition.

II- Short acting anti-muscarinic bronchodilators, such as Ipratropium bromide monohydrate. Ipratropium bromide monohydrate blocks muscarinic cholinergic receptors, resulting in bronchodilation. Aerosol inhalation of ipratropium has a maximum effect 30-60 minutes after use, and duration of action of 3-6 hours. Ipratropium bromide can be used to provide short-term relief of asthma symptoms.

B-Preventers:

Preventer medications are primarily, Corticosteroids such as beclometasone dipropionate, budesonide, fluticasone propionate, mometasone furoate. A preventer is normally taken regularly, even if there are no Asthma symptoms and usually taken long-term.

When appropriate preventer is used consistently as prescribed over time it is believed to prevent/control inflammation in the airways, reducing acute episodes of Asthma even if the patient comes into contact with a known Asthma trigger, and preventing long-term lung damage.

Inhaled corticosteroids do not normally have the same bioavailability as oral systemic corticosteroids; hence, the risk of potential side effects is believed to be substantially reduced.

C-Symptoms controllers

Symptoms controllers are primarily long acting beta$_2$agonists, such as salmeterol xinafoate and formoterol fumarate. There is also a long acting anti-muscarinic such as tiotropium bromide.

The increased lipophilicity of long acting bronchodilators (LABAs) compared to short acting bronchodilators (relievers) leads to prolonged retention in the lung tissues. LABAs have duration of bronchodilation at least 12 hours after single use, thus LABAs relieve asthma symptoms for longer periods.

Long-acting beta$_2$-agonists (LABAs) or long acting anti-muscarinic should not be used as monotherapy for long-term control of Asthma, they are usually added to a corticosteroid preventer therapy and it is currently not recommended to use Asthma controllers to treat acute symptoms or exacerbations of Asthma according to current guidelines of the American and British Thoracic Societies.

D-Asthma prophylaxis

Sodium cromoglicate and nedocromils are believed to inhibit mediators release from inflammatory cells. Sodium cromoglicate or nedocromil may be of value as prophylaxis in Asthma with an allergic basis. Nedocromil may be also of some benefit in the prophylaxis of exercise -induced Asthma according to published literature.

3-Aerosol inhalers

An aerosol is a suspension of liquid or solid particles in a carrier gas. Aerosol inhalers can be divided into three groups:

3.1-Pressurised metered dose inhalers (pMDI)

pMDI device, delivers a measured amount of medication into the lungs in the form of a short burst of aerosolized medicine. The pressurised metered dose inhaler (pMDI) device was discovered in 1955 by the American Doctor George Maison. Dr Maison realised that storing Asthma drugs inside a pressurised canister meant, they could be easily expelled into the lungs with one button push (figures 6 and 7).

In pMDIs, the drug is dissolved or suspended in a propellant under pressure, when activated a valve system releases a metered volume of drug and propellant. Common environmentally friendly propellants currently used in Asthma inhalers is (1,1,1,2-tetrafluoroethane usually written as HFA-134a). pMDIs may still have the word CFC free, which means that they do not contain chlorofluorocarbons. Chlorofluorocarbons (CFCS) propellants are believed to cause ozone depletion or a hole in ozone layer.

The pMDI is one of the most commonly used device in management of Asthma, pMDIs can unfortunately be difficult for some patients to use and even with repeated demonstration and assessment some patients will still find co-ordination of the whole technique challenging, failing to master it despite repetition. [6 Babies], young children, or adult patients with co-ordination problem normally use the pMDIs with a spacer device.

Normally when a company produces a new inhaler device for Asthma medication, the inhaler device is patented as well as the dosage form/s delivered from that device to the patent holder. The patent holder can use the same type of device for delivery of different types of inhaled Asthma medications. The patent for some inhalation devices have expired which means that other companies can use similar devices for their products. For some of the inhalation devices described here the patent has expired which means the same type of device can be used freely by pharmaceutical companies other than the original patent holder. An inhaler, which still patented to a pharmaceutical company, is considered an intellectual property of the company.

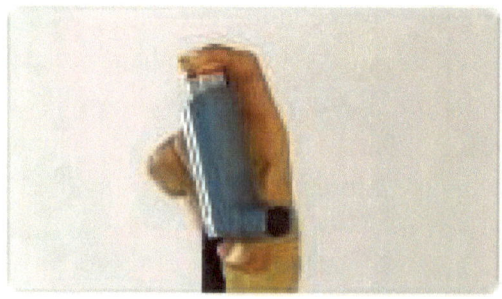

Fig 6. Pressurised metered dose inhaler (pMDIs) or puffer

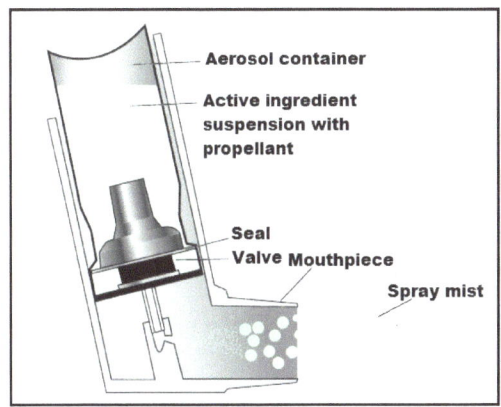

Fig 7. Illustrated cross-section through a pressurised metered-dose inhaler (pMDI)

The correct use of pMDI requires co-ordination of depressing the inhaler and breathing thus the use of this inhaler requires good hand lung co-ordination. Correct breathing pattern for pMDIs is deep slow breath and holding the breath as long as possible. Good hand lung co-ordination helps to deliver more of the correct sized particles to the alveolar region, thus improve efficiency of inhaled aerosol.

Pressurised metered dose inhaler (pMDI) with spacer

The effective use of pMDI requires good hand breath co-ordination. Some patients just cannot achieve the required co-ordination in particular young children. In the case of inability to manage the required co-ordination, a spacer device may be used with pMDIs (figures 8 and 9).

A spacer is a plastic or metal container, with a mouthpiece at one end and a hole for the aerosol inhaler at the other.

17

Spacer devices remove the need for coordination between Actuation of a pressurized metered-dose inhaler and Inhalation. The spacer device reduces the velocity of the Aerosol and subsequent impaction on the oropharynx and Allows more time for evaporation of the propellant so that a larger proportion of the particles can be inhaled and deposited in the lungs.

Pressurised metered dose inhalers (pMDIs) are the only inhaler devices, which could be used with spacers. Spacer can help patients, who have difficulty with press and breathe inhaler use, Some spacer devices are also outfitted with an audible flow signal that will sound if the patient inhales too quickly.

Some spacers can be used with facemasks. Very young children may require a mask to ensure as much asthma medication as possible is breathed into their lungs. Facemasks are also useful for adults who have difficulty taking their medication without a facemask.

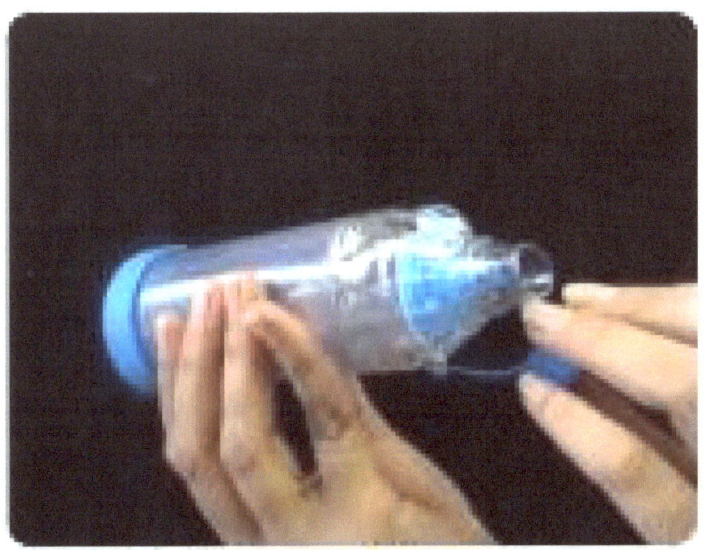

Fig 8. Aerochamber® adult Spacer with a mouthpiece

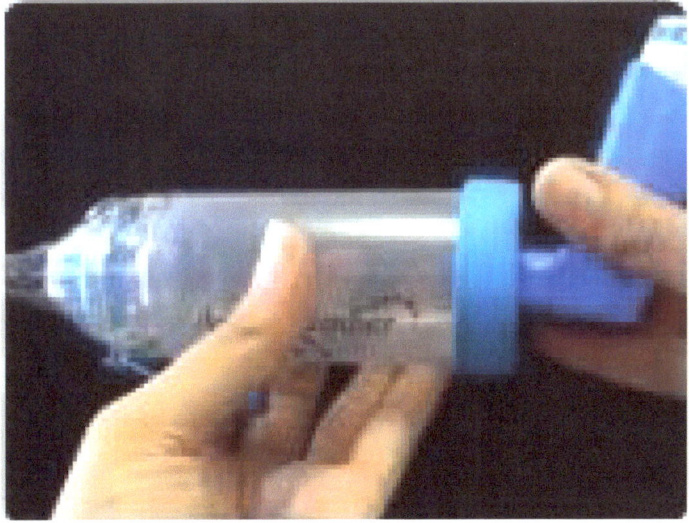

Fig 9. pMDI attached to a spacer

Young children should use pMDI with a spacer and a facemask and then move into a spacer with a mouthpiece when they are able to, as directed by the prescriber.[3] Spacers can help adult patients who have difficulty with use of press and breathe inhalers.

Spacers are also used in order to reduce potential for side effects from medication such as the use of corticosteroids containing inhalers. The use of spacers is recommended for the delivery of inhaled corticosteroids in all age groups in the USA[3], and for all children under 15 years in the U.K.[5]

3.2-Breathe-activated pMDIs

The metered medication dose from this type of pressurised inhalers, is released when the patient breathes in. Two brands of breathe-activated pMDIs are available, Autohaler® and Easi-breathe®. A metered dose from breathe-acivated inhalers is fired by a spring, which is triggered by airflow at the onset of inpiration, this removes the need for hand breath co-ordination. Spacers should not be used with Breathe-activated pMDIs

Qvar50® **Autohaler®**, contains beclometasone di propionate is an example of breath activated inhaler which still under patent. In QVAR® Autohaler®, the patient load required dose, ready for inhalation by raising the lever on the top of the inhaler, then activates the inhaler by breathing in. The autohaler device makes quite a sharp, loud noise that some individuals may stop breathing when the drug is released (figures 10 and 11).

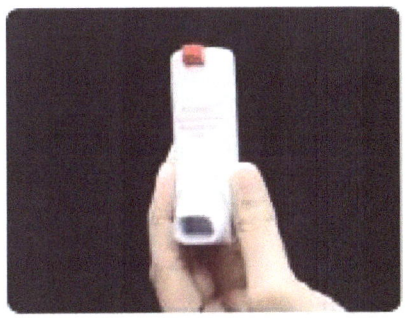

Fig 10. QVAR® Autohaler®.

The Autohaler® is activated by breath; therefore, the use of the Autohaler® does not require hand-breath coordination to inhale the aerosol medicine. This can be very useful for people having trouble with the timing and co-ordination technique needed for pMDI devices. The device is such that the medication is delivered automatically during inspiration without the need for the patient to co-ordinate with inhalation.

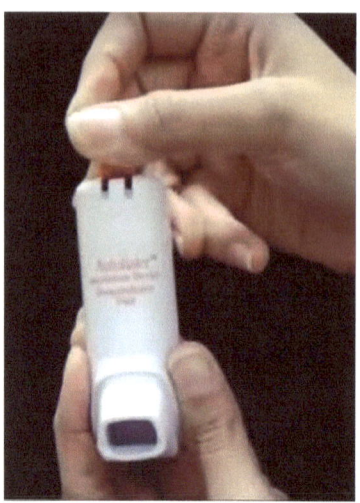

Fig 11. The lever on the top of the QVAR® autohaler® is raised, ready for inhalation

3.3-Non-pressurised aerosol inhalers

Spiriva® Respimat® inhaler is a hand held, pocket sized oral inhalation device that uses mechanical energy generated by a compressed spring, not a propellant to generate a slow moving aerosol cloud of medication from a metered volume of the drug solution (figures 12 and 13).

A twist of the inhaler base compresses a spring and the required dose is moved into the dosing chamber. When the dose-release button is pressed, the energy released from the spring forces the solution through the uniblock and a slow moving cloud is released from two jets at precise angles (figure 14).

The aerosol generated by the device also has smaller particle size than that generated by conventional pMDI, resulting in superior deposition in the lower airways[6].

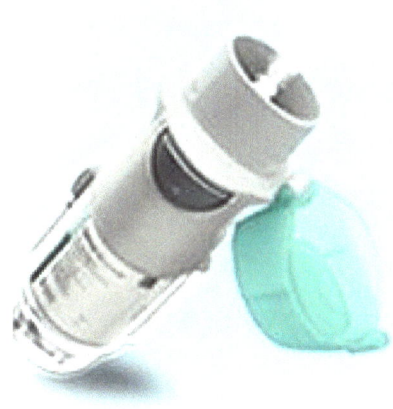

Fig 12. Spiriva® Respimat®

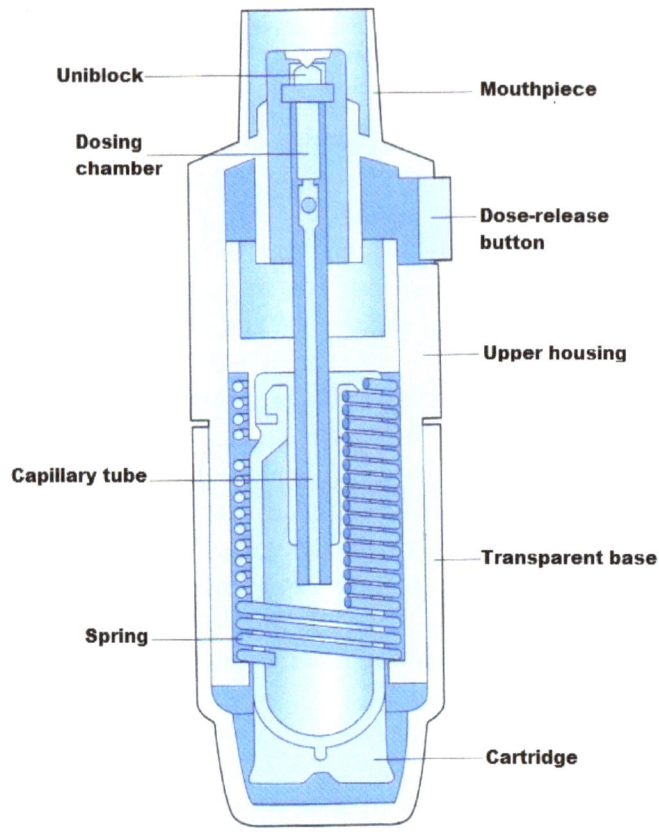

Fig 13. A cross-section of respimat® inhaler

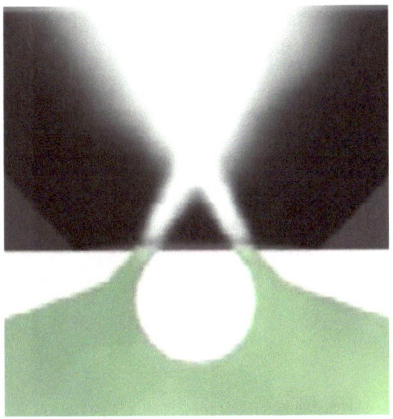

Fig 14. Aerosol generation in respimat® inhaler.

4-Dry powder inhalers

Dry powder inhalers (DPIs) are portable inspiratory flow driven devices that deliver dry powder formulations of inhaled drugs to the lungs. Each DPI requires a specific priming procedure, the obervance of which is critical in making the drug available for inhalation. Therefore clear instructions to the user is mandatory.

Inspiratory volume and flows generated by the patient are the main factors that determine the drug delivery to the lungs. Dry powder inhalers require deeper stronger breath in. The minimum inspiratory flow required varies greatly depending on the specific type of device used.

Inspiratory flow measurement using the inspiratory flow meter can be useful in the selection and efficient use of inhalers. Inspiratory flow meters can also be used in the measurement of inspiratory capability of asthma patients and in the area of inhaler technique training (figure 15).

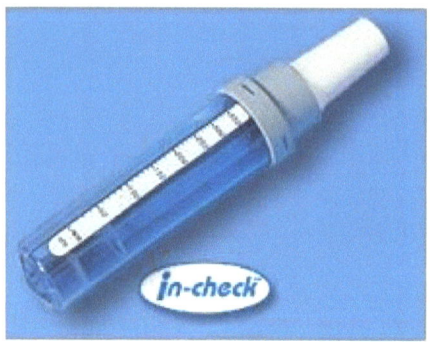

Fig 15. Inspiratory flow meter

One thing to note about and inspiratory flow meter versus expiratory flow meter is the plastic. In the inspiratory flow meter, it is a clear plastic versus the opaque expiratory flow meters. This is, so that, the user can look inside to see if there are any broken parts that the patient could possibly inhale.

When using dry powder inhalers, it is important that the patient exhales away from the device to prevent introducing humidity into the medication or blowing away the dose. Dry powder inhalers may be easier to use than pMDIs, if patient struggles with co-ordination. Hand-breath co-ordination is not required for dry powder inhalers. Spacers should not be used with dry powder inhalers.

4.1-Multidose dry powder inhalers

Dry powder inhalers which contain multiunit doses in blister ready for inhalation for example Diskus / Accuhaler and Elitra contain multidoses in blisters. Turbohalers, Flexhalers and Twisthalers are examples of dry powder inhalers, which contain the multidoses in a bulk powder reservoir inside the inhalers.

Diskus/Accuhaler

Diskus/Accuhaler is a a multidose Dry powder inhaler (DPI) with drug in foil blisters, the blister contains 60 doses of medication in a lactose based carrier. Many Asthma medications are available in Accuhaler/Diskus inhaler devices (figure 16). Inside the diskus or accuhaler one wheel contains 60 doses of powder medication individually wrapped in blisters on a foil strip. The foil blisters protects the medication from humidity and provide a relatively consistent dose over a wide range of flow rates. The Accuhaler has a dose counter, the dose counter counts down from 60-0, the last five doses are in red.

Common errors in using the Accuhaler include; failure to breath in deeply, with enough force to inhale powdered formulation.

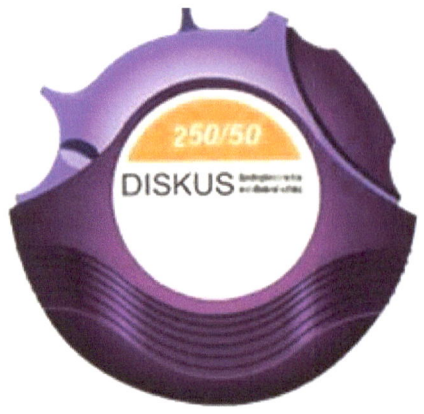

Fig 16. Accuhaler/Diskus

Diskus is a DPI. DPIs do not use propellants like pressurized Metered dose inhalers (pMDI), so they do not require hand-breath co-ordination or slow and deep breathing technique. Your breathing should be Quick and Deep enough to inhale the powdered medicine from the inhaler device.

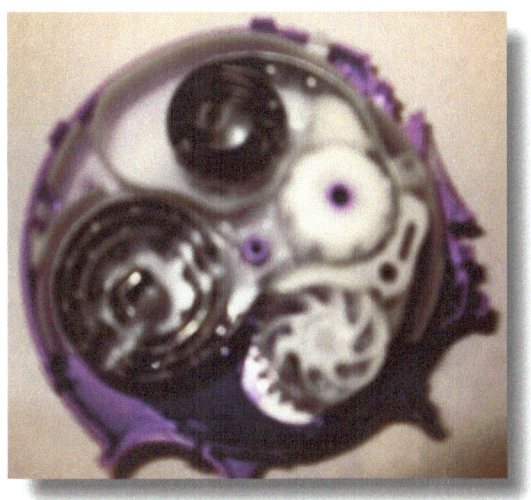

Fig 17. A view inside the diskus/accuhaler. on one coil blisters of medicinal powder, once the content of a blister is inhaled the empty blister moves into a nother coil of emptied blisters.

Relvar® Ellipta®

Relvar® Ellipta® has moderate resistance to airflow and can hold one or two blister strips, with each blister containing a sealed single dose of medication. Mono therapies can be delivered by the single-strip configuration and, in the two-strip configuration, one dose from each strip can be aerosolized simultaneously to allow combination therapies to be delivered, which enables the formulations for each product to be developed individually, since they are stored separately until the point of administration. There are three principal operating steps to administer a dose: open, inhale, close (figure 18).

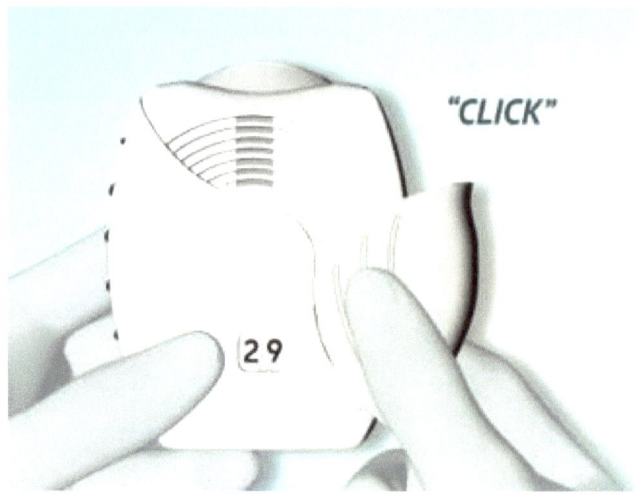

Fig 18. Relvar® Ellipta® is a combination of two medicines-
an inhaled corticosteroid (ICS) fluticasone furoate, and a
long-acting beta2-adrenergic agonist (LABA) called
vilanterol.

Turbohalers®

Turbohalers are dry powder inhalers which contain multi-
dose of bulk powder in the inhaler, individual doses are
loaded into dosing compartment prior to inhalation by the
patient. There are other bulk dry powder inhalers such as
Clickhaler®, Easyhaler® Twisthaler, Flexhaler (figure 19).

The content of the Turbohaler is either in the form of a fine
powder of medicine only, example Bricanyl® Turbohaler, or
fine powder of medicine and lactose, example symbicort®
Turbohaler. The device contains a number of doses of
drug, which is stored in bulk powder in a reservoir. As the

inhaler is rotated as directed, one metered dose is loaded on the the inhalation disc and this is inhaled by the patient.

Humidity is a concern with DPIs because of the potential for powder clumping and reduced dispersal of fine particle mass.[8] Humidity can originate from the ambient air or from patient exhalation into the mouthpiece. DPI design influences the effect of humidity. Multi-dose bulk powder reservoirs (eg, Turbuhaler) are more vulnerable than devices that use blister packs (eg, Diskus) in which the Powder is protected.[9]

Some Turbohalers require an inspiratory flow > 60 L/min to effectively de-aggregate the powder, that flow cannot always be achieved by children and patients with severe airflow obstruction.[10] Turbohaler® will rattle if it is shaken, even when there is no more medication inside the inhaler, the rattling is due to the desicator rather than the medication.

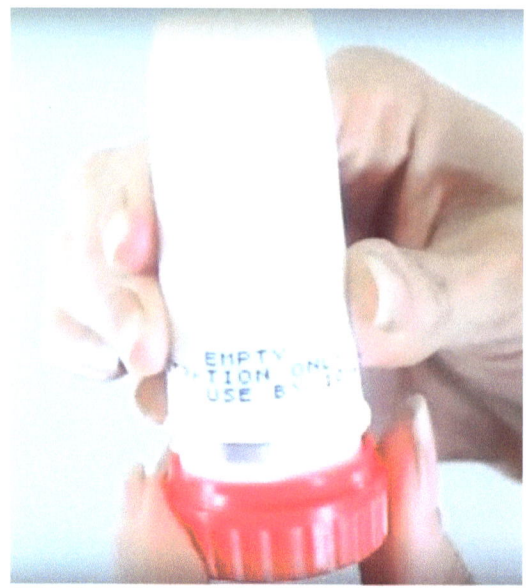

Fig 19. Turbohaler®

4.2-Unit-dose DPIs

Unit dose DPIs are designed to use individual dose units normally capsules, the individual dose units need to be loaded by the patient before taking each each dose, examples of this type of dry powder inhaler are Spiriva® Handihaler®, and Foradil® Aerolizer® . Spiriva®Handihaler® is a single dose DPI device. It delivers medicine in the form of dry powder contained in a capsule. The capsule dosage form contains a dry powder formulation of tiotropium intended for inhalation only with the Spiriva®Handihaler® device (figure 20 and 21).

In order to inhale the capsule content, a single capsule is placed into a loose-fitting rotor inside the device. The capsule is pierced by metal needle on the sides of the capsule. Inhaled air flow through the device causes the rotor to rotate rapidly causing the powder to move to the capsule walls and out into the inspired air. It is important to explain to the patient that the capsule cannot be taken orally, and should only be inhaled using the supplied handihaler.

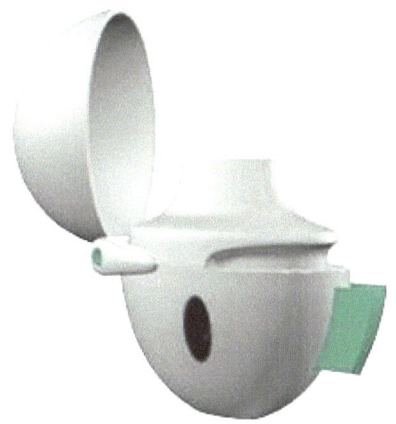

Fig 20. Spiriva® HandiHaler®

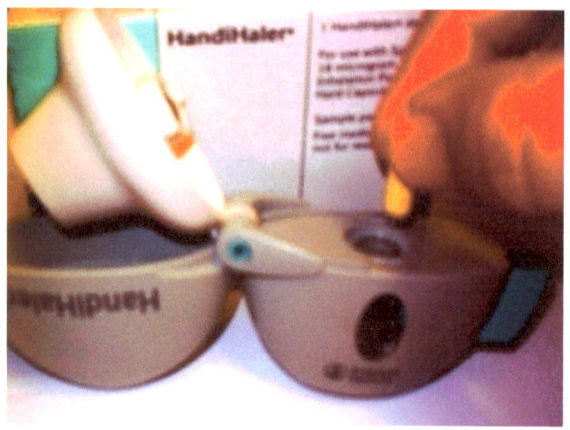

Fig 21. Loading dose into Spiriva® Handihaler®

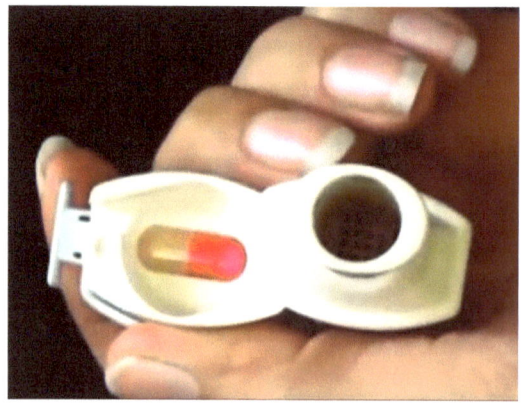

Fig 22. Foradil® Aerolizer®

5-Patient education and inhaler training

Patients may find it challenging to take their Asthma inhaler medication as prescribed, differentiate between their maintenance and rescue inhalers and correctly operate their inhalers. Sestini *et al* [11.] Conducted an observational study of 1,305 patients on their use of pMDIs and DPIs. With both types of inhalers, misuse was significantly and equally associated with older age, less education, and less instruction by healthcare personnel.

Asthma patients should be advised that by using their prescribed device/s properly and taking medication as prescribed, they will be getting the best chance of reducing Asthma symptoms and living well with Asthma. Inhalation devices which contain preventer medications should be used regularly not as required, and they normally take a week or longer to start improving symptoms after initial first use.

Sometimes a patient could not use a particular prescribed inhaler device. If the patient finds the device tricky to use, the pharmacist or local Asthma nurse can help him/her use the device or, advice the prescriber to replace it with alternative inhalation device, which the patient can use.

In order to use any inhalation device, the patient must be sitting or standing in an upright position prior to using their inhaler; Following inhalation the individual should hold their breath for 10 seconds or as long as possible prior to exhalation.

With respect to quick relief inhaler or rescue medicine, all patients should be given the following advices; Carry your quick-relief inhaler with you at all times in case you need it. If your child has asthma, make sure that anyone caring for him or her has the child's quick-relief medicines, including staff at the child's school. They should understand when and how to use these medicines and when to seek medical care for your child. You should not use quick-relief medicines in place of prescribed long-term control medicines. Quick-relief medicines do not reduce inflammation.

Inhaled corticosteroids are the preferred medicine for long-term control of asthma. They are the most effective option for long-term relief of the inflammation and swelling that make your airways sensitive to certain inhaled substances. One common side effect from inhaled corticosteroids is a mouth infection called thrush. You might be able to use a spacer or holding chamber on your inhaler to avoid thrush. These devices attach to your inhaler. They help prevent the medicine from landing in your mouth or on the back of your throat.

Patients using steroid containing inhalers should rinse their mouth and spit out immediately after using their steroid inhaler in order to reduce the chances of getting local side effects like oral thrush. If the patient has dentures these should be removed and cleaned to ensure any particles under the plate are removed.

It is recommended to develop a personalized management plan for asthma patients. Asthma management plan normally includes: ways to avoid asthma triggers, medications to prevent symptoms as well as medications to use for quick relief of flare-ups, in addition to asthma action plan to identify when the patient is doing well and when they need to seek help.[2]

Inhaler training
Ideally, Asthma management would begin with the doctor providing the basis of disease care and management, with nurses and pharmacists providing supplementary education, reviewing and teaching improved inhaler use. It has been demonstrated that the majority of healthcare professionals cannot demonstrate correct inhaler use to their patients, it is

not therefore not surprising that patients are mostly unable to demonstrate good inhaler technique, this results in poorer control of asthma, hospitalisation and increased healthcare costs.[2]

Not only various patients' characteristics but also the device that patients use to inhale the medicine has an effect on correct inhalation technique. Many patients derive incomplete benefit from their inhaled medication because they do not use their inhaler devices correctly or they fail to maintain the correct inhaler technique. This is clearly one of the major limitations in treating Asthma. Further, there is evidence that the use of multiple inhaler types confuses the patient and increases the risk of errors in their inhaler use. In order to deal with it, there is a clear need for specific inhaler technique education and training of patients. Asthma patients need to be shown and trained on how to use inhaler devices properly. An appropriately trained person, usually an asthma nurse, pharmacist, or a doctor may demonstrate correct inhaler technique together with explanation of the importance for each step of the instructions.

Inhaler training strategy

Two inhaler training strategies are normally considered– the brief intervention and the teach-to-goal methods were investigated by Press *et al* [12], with the teach-to-goal method having been found to be the most effective method overall. This approach involves repeated demonstration and allowing the patient to demonstrate it back thus enhancing the memory on allowing the patient to "teach it back" to the healthcare professional. The brief intervention approach involves brief verbal instruction on correct technique, with a physical demonstration, which is repeated over time as needed. A study by Cordina et al [13], indicated that pharmacist intervention in monitoring asthma management in general was well received by the patients involved and had good influence on the patients' inhaler technique.

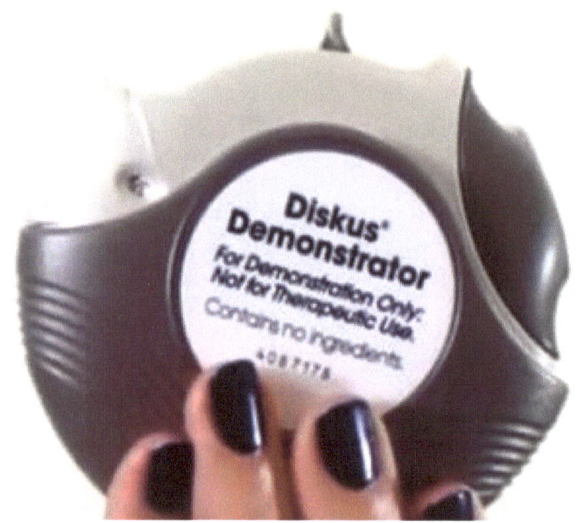

Fig 23. Placebo Disckus/Accuhaler

Main benefits of using Placebo inhalers:

1-The trainer can demonstrate the technique for the patient using their own placebo inhaler
2-The patient can make several attempts at perfecting their technique
3-If the patient is unable to perfect the technique of one device, they can attempt alternative devices to assist in choosing the most appropriate.
4-It is essential that healthcare professionals have easy access to placebo inhaler devices to assess a patient's overall inhaler technique, since these will allow the patient

to be assessed on the priming, positioning and coordination of the device.

5-Many centres advice that placebo inhalers should be 'single-patient use' only, since there is a theoretical risk of infection when using placebo inhalers among patients.

Concluding remarks

Objective measures of lung function are normally used in order to assess the severity of asthma and to monitor the course of therapy.

Asthmatic patients need to avoid or eliminate factors that precipitate asthma symptoms or exacerbations.

Direct delivery of medication to the lungs is a major component in the treatment of asthma. After prescribing appropriate therapy, correct inhaler technique is a cornerstone of achieving adequate therapy.

Different inhaler types are currently available with differences in dose priming and dose inhalation techniques required. Optimal inhaler technique allows maximal drug delivery to the lungs and so improving symptom control.

Regardless of the type of inhaler device prescribed, patients are unlikely to use inhalers correctly unless they receive clear instructions, including physical demonstrations.

Successful training in inhaler technique depends upon effective communication of proper technique and its purpose, and monitoring to ensure that the skills have been learned and retained.

It is desirable that the range of drugs prescribed to an individual is delivered through similar devices, within the availability of drug/device combinations.

6-Self assessment questions; Multiple choice

questions, select the most appropriate answer.

Q1: A 13 year old child is prescribed clenil modulite 50 (beclometasone 50 micrograms/metered inhalation dose) and a spacer device.   The mum asks you why did the prescriber prescribe the spacer device as her son has been using ventolin evohaler without spacer for two years without spacer.   What would be your answer?

A-It could be a mistake.

B-Do not use the spacer.

C-Use the spacer with clenil, to reduce side effects.

D-Use the spacer with ventolin evohaler to reduce side effects.

Q2: A 30 year old patient is prescribed clenil modulite 100 (beclometasone 100 micrograms/metered inhalation dose) inhaler together with a ventolin evohaler and a spacer to use with clenil modulite inhaler, the patient asks your advice about over the counter medicine for oral thrush which he gets regularly, what advice would you offer the patient which may reduce frequency of oral thrush?

A-Do not use the spacer with clenil modulite.

B-Use the spacer with ventolin it might help.

C-Use both inhalers with spacer it might help.

D-Carry on using clenil modulite with spacer, and rinse your mouth with water and spit out after use.

Q3:A 38 year old patient is prescribed ventolin evohaler (salbutamol 100 micrograms/metered inhalation dose), two puffs up to four times daily if required, the patient asks, can she inhale the two puffs at the same time.

A-Yes as long as she hold her breath twice as long.

B-No it is better to wait about 15 minutes between before inhaling the second dose.

C-No it is better to 30 minutes.

D-No, current advice, it is best to wait about one minute between one puff and the other.

Q4:A patient is prescribed ventolin evohaler (salbutamol 100 micrograms/metered inhalation dose) and clenil modulite 100 beclometasone 100 micrograms/metered inhalation dose), the patient sometimes needs to use both at the same time, which one of the following statements is correct:

A-Use clenil modulite first and wait one minute before using ventolin.

B-Use ventolin inhaler first,and wait 9 minutes before using clenil modulite.

C-Use ventolin first and wait 4 minutes before using clenil modulite.

D-Use ventolin first and wait one minute before using clenil modulite.

Q5: Which one of the following inhaler devices contains a reliever medication:

A-Serevent   50   accuhaler   (salmetrol   50 micrograms/inhalation dose).

B-QVAR 100 autohaler beclometasone dipropionate/ 100 micrograms inhalation dose) .

C-Flixotide   50   inhaler   (fluticasone   propionate/50 micrograms inhalation dose).

D-Airomir 100 autohaler (salbutamol/100 micrograms inhalation dose).

Q6:A patient asks you how often does he need to replace the spacer, which of the following is the most appropriate answer:

A-Replace every month and sooner if it damaged.

B-Every three months and sooner if it is damaged.

C-Usually every year but follow manufacturers advice.

D-You only change it if itis broken.

Q7:You receive a valid legal prescription for a two year old child for ventolin evohaler (salbutamol/100 micrograms inhalation dose), the dose is one or two puffs as required up to four times daily, the child's mum told you this is the first time the child is prescribed ventolin evohaler, what item is missing from the prescription?

A-The prescription should have a preventer.

B-The prescription should have spacer with a mouthpiece.

C-The prescription should have a controller inhaler.

D-The prescription should have a suitable spacer for the child's age.

Q8: Which one of the following inhalers can not be used with a spacer device:

A-Flixotide   100   inhaler (fluticasone   propionate/100 micrograms inhalation dose).

B-Seretide   50   inhaler   (fluticasone   propionate   50 micrograms and salmeterol 25 micrograms/ metered dose inhalation).

C-Serevent 25 inhaler (salmetrol 25 micrograms/inhalation dose).

D-Salamol   100   easi-breathe   (salbutamol   100 micrograms/inhalation dose).

Q9: A 9 year old child is prescribed clenil modulite 50 inhaler   (50   micrograms   beclometasone dipropionate/dose), with suitable spacer for the first time. Which is the correct course of action you should take:

A-Tell mum the child does not need spacer.

B-Dispense QVAR 50 inhaler.

C-Dispense Clenil modulite 50 with advice.

D-Confirm with prescriber specific brand required.

Q10: Which one of the following dry powder inhalers can be used with a spacer device

A-Serevent accuhaler.

B-Seretide accuhaler.

C-Symbicort Turbohaler.

D-None.

Answers

Q1 -C

Q2 -D

Q3 -D

Q4 -D

Q5 -D

Q6 -C

Q7 -D

Q8 -D

Q9 –C

Q10 -D

7-References

1-Al-Jahdali H, Ahmed A, Al-Harbi A, Khan M, Baharoon S, Bin Saleh S, et al. Improper inhaler technique is associated with poor asthma control and frequent emergency department visits. Allergy, Asthma and clinical immunology. 2013; 9: 8-14.

2-Global initiative for Global strategy for asthma management and prevention, 2012. Available from http://www.ginasthma.org/documents/4. Accessed on 18/03/16.

3-Expert panel report 3: Guidelines for the diagnosis and management of asthma. Bethesda, Maryland: National Institutes of health, National Asthma Education and prevention program; 207, NIH publication No.08-4051. http://www.nhlbi.nih.gov/guidelines/asthma/asthdln.pdf. Accessed 18/03/2016.

4-British National Formulary (BNF), 09/2013, 66th ed. Pharmaceutical Press, London.

5-Virchow JC, Crompton GK, Dal Negro R, Pedersen S, Magnan A, Sedenberg J, Barnes PJ. Importance of inhaler devices in the management of airway disease. Respiratory Medicine. 2008; 102 (1): 10-19.

6-Hess DR. Aerosol delivery devices in the treatment of asthma. Respiratory care. 2008; 53 (6): 699-723.

7-JVD Pallen. Peak inspiratory flow through diskus and turbohaler, measured by means of a peak inspiratory flow meter (in check dial®). Respiratory medicine. 2003; 97: 285-289.

8-Maggi L, Bruni R, Conte U. Influence of the moisture on the performance of a new dry powder inhaler. Int J Pharm 1999; 177 (1): 83-91.

9-Rau JL. Practical problems with aerosol therapy in COPD. Respir Care. 2006; 51 (2): 158-172.

10-De Boer AH, Winter HMI, Lerk CF. Inhalation characteristics and their effect on in-vitro drug delivery from dry powder inhalers. Int J Pharm Pharmacol. 1996; 130: 231-244.

11-Sestini P, Cappiello V, Aliani M, et al. Prescription bias and factors associated with improper use of inhalers. J Aerosol Med. 2006; 19 (2): 127-136.

12-Press VG, Arora VM, Shah LM, Lewis SL, Charbeneau J, Naureckas ET, et al. Teaching the use of respiratory inhalers to hospitalisation patients with asthma or COPD: A randomized trial. Journal of General Internal medicine. 2012; 27 (10): 1317-1325.

13-Cordina M, McElnay JC, Hughes CM. Assessment of a community pharmacy-based program for patients with asthma. Pharmacotherapy. 2001; 21 (10): 1196-1203.

14-British National Formulary for children, (BNFC), 2013-2014, Pharmaceutical Press, London.

15-Micallef LA. A review of the metered dose inhaler technique in asthmatic and COPD patients. Malta medical journal. 2015; 27 (01): 22-28.

16-Dolovich MB, Aherns RC, Hess DR, Anderson P, Dhard R, Rau JL, et al. Device selection and outcomes of aerosol therapy: evidence-based guidelines: American college of chest physicians/ American College Asthma, Allergy, and Immunology. Chest. 2005; 127: 335-371.

17-Kips JC, Pauwels RA, Long-acting inhaled beta$_2$ agonist therapy in asthma. Am J respire crit care med 2001; 164 (6): 923-32.

18-Grossman J., The evolution of inhaler technology. Journal of asthma 31, (1994), 55-64.

19-Chrystyn H. Is inhalation rate important for a dry powder inhaler? Using the In-Check Dial to identify these rates. Respir Med 2003;97(2):181-7.